Headache Cures Made Easy

How To Heal Migraines & Headaches Forever The Natural Way

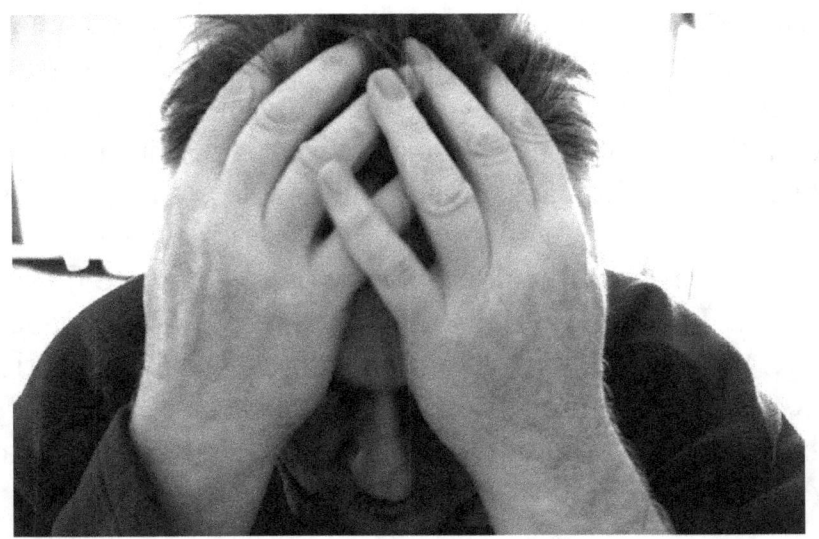

NOTES TO THE READER

From The Author

Thank you for taking the time to read this book. As an author, I understand the importance of creating books which my readers will find both enjoyable and informative. If you have the time and feel generous, please don't hesitate to leave an honest review of this book.........Dr Brad Turner.

Contents

Introduction

What can cause headaches and when is it necessary to see a doctor? Headaches definitely should not be underestimated. In some cases, they significantly reduce quality of life and may even be accompanied by a serious illness. The group of possible headaches is very large; some may be subject of pathological processes in the brain, and then there are so-called functional headaches. Headaches can also be caused by an excessive use of some analgesics – painkillers - but other drugs with known side effects can also cause trouble. This condition may be accompanied by other diseases of the head or neck, and pain may also appear in connection with certain medical procedures. Headaches are not just a problem of hypochondriacs and privileged hysteric women. This is a real disease, which is described by the International Classification of Diseases.

Headache as a symptom may be accompanied by common diseases, but on the other hand, it may also be a life-threatening condition. Pain warns us that something is not right with our body. Acute pain is usually a signal for indicating imbalance of our body´s workings. Perception and pain management are concerned with sensory nerve fibers and their endings. The brain itself does not have these fibers, and therefore the brain is not able to experience pain. Headaches as known by most people have their origins outside the cranial cavity. Skin, muscles, ligaments, surface of bones, eyes, and teeth are richly interwoven with sensitive nerve fibers and these can be a source of intense pain.

The cause of pain can be a variety of pathological processes, for example tumors, stroke, bleeding, or conditions that arise after injuries. If the pain occurs suddenly or unexpectedly, when half of the head hurts or a person constantly feels pressure pain in which he or she is unable to do anything and each movement increases the pain, the person should see a doctor. Conventional medications will not help.

The largest group, about 75%, constitute the so-called primary headaches. Their formation is not contingent upon any other condition. The most famous of them is definitely the migraine, but the most common is the so-called tension-type headache (headache of excessive mental strain). Primary headaches that occur with diabetes, obesity, high blood pressure, heart attacks, or strokes are sometimes called "civilization diseases". 93% of men and 99% of women suffer one of the above mentioned headaches. Signs of migraine can occur at any age. Seizures usually begin in childhood or in adolescence. It affects boys more often, but the ratio moves "in favor" of girls at puberty. If the person repeatedly suffers headaches, look for a doctor. Probably he will tell you that everything is alright, but if not, he will send the patient for further examination. Each headache should be properly examined. Headache can occur due to a variety of reasons.

Primary headaches such as migraines are caused by neurochemical changes in the brain. Secondary headaches arise as a result of another disease, such as head trauma, brain tumors, pressure changes in the cranial cavity, infection, drugs, etc. A number of systemic diseases and disorders can cause headaches. These include high blood pressure, anemia, heart disease, lung cancer, sleep disorders, or AIDS. If a person suffers from headaches, he/she should look at the nature of the pain (dull, sharp, etc.), pain location, time aspects of pain (how long it takes, in which part of the day) associated factors (linked to the weather), and presence or absence of neurological symptoms (weakness, numbness, etc.). These factors help determine the type of headache and its treatment. First steps necessary for successful control over headaches are correct diagnosis and early treatment. It is very important to distinguish primary headache from secondary headache.

The norm for determining the type of headache is the classification system of IHS (International Headache Society). The system divides headaches into two main groups - the primary headaches, categories 1-4, and secondary headaches, categories 5 – 14. Primary headaches have no known organic base, which could be seen using CT or MRI. The only problem is pain. Therefore, primary headaches are classified according to their symptoms. In the group of secondary headache pain there is an organic base, so in these groups can be found classification of various types of headaches, based on knowledge of the causes of medical problems.

CHAPTER 1

THE FACTS ABOUT HEADACHES

The most common type of headache is so-called tension-type or vasomotor pain, forming nearly 90 percent of all headaches. They are very strong and can return often. Migraine is a throbbing pain that usually affects only one half of the head; attacks can take hours or even days, and often are preceded by warning signs. There is still not a simple definition of tension-type headache. It can be characterized as a dull pain that is associated with tiredness, which is often preceded by stress.

The pain in tension-type headache is often located in the front of the cranial cavity. It is dull, stable, and of fluctuating intensity. Its onset is usually gradual and often occurs at night or afternoon. Patients often complain of a feeling of pressure, discomfort when combing, stiffness in the neck muscles, feeling of a clamping ring around the head, swelling, and sometimes a feeling of pressure in the head. Actuator can be not only stress alone, but also repeated conflicts and even expectation of conflicts. Present is sometimes depression, and especially common in chronic conditions are sleep disorders. Subjective difficulties are not worsened by physical activity or alcohol. In the physical examination, we can find an increased sensitivity to muscle palpation. We need to eliminate possible causes of secondary headache.

Basically, tension headache is persistent pain throughout the head or in tender points located mainly on the neck and upper teeth. Accumulated tension-type headache is intense throbbing pain on one side of the head, which occurs several times during a day and in some cases for several months. A migraine is an intense throbbing pain, at first near to one eye or during sleep, then across the middle of the head or the entire head. Early warning signs include colored circles below the eyes, wavy contours of the visual field, ringing in the ears, dizziness, sweating, fatigue, swelling of the face and irritability.

The exact cause of headaches is not known yet, but it is believed that stimulants are spasms of the arteries that supply the brain with blood. This may be due to low levels of serotonin in the brain. Migraines tend to be hereditary diseases and women tend to be more prone to them than men.

CHAPTER 2

PRIMARY HEADACHES

Migraine is a chronic disease characterized by attacks of throbbing headache (mostly on one half of the head). Pain lasts 4-72 hours, often associated with nausea, vomiting, anxiety, and hypersensitivity to light and sound. With an increase of physical activity, the pain worsens. Migraine attack is not just pain.

An attack has several stages. Primary stage: Several hours or days before seizure, there are changes of mood, irritability, decreased concentration, and increased urinary frequency. The next stage is the "aura". It is observed by only 15-20% of patients. Aura can be visual (flashing and waving in the visual field), sensitive, sensory, motoric or mixed. Then there is a stage of pain. Headache is usually moderate to high intensity, mostly localized in the temple area and around the eye. It is a throbbing pain, sharp, unpleasant, which is accentuated by physical strain. Untreated migraine lasts 4-72 hours and then spontaneously subsides. Finally, there is a last stage. After the pain, the patient is often tired, and has difficulties with concentrating.

Additional factors may be stress, change of weather, change in hormonal situation by women or lack of sleep. Physical activity worsens migraine pain. Migraine headaches are mostly one-sided, or sometimes both and sometimes alternating sides. There is no test or examination which confirms the diagnosis of migraine. The cause of a pressure headache can be stress. It is caused by muscle contraction. We can speak about mild pain, which affects the whole head.

They can take different lengths of time, but nausea is absent and physical activity does not make pain worse.

SECONDARY HEADACHES

Post-traumatic pain occurs after head injuries. It can be accompanied by dizziness, tiredness, and bad concentration and memory skills. Increase or decrease of inner cranial pressure can cause headaches, nausea, vomiting, and blurred vision. Infection (meningitis, encephalitis) causes pain throughout the head. Diseases such as ischemia, hemorrhage, and vasculitis do not cause headaches. Brain tumors are the cause of headaches in less than 1% of cases. They show by higher pain intensity, and pain persists even after analgesics. Pain increases when coughing and sneezing. By the secondary headache, patient usually has a high temperature.

Eye pain may be associated with increased eye strain (work with a computer, watching TV, reading). Headaches may also occur in some systemic diseases, notably the flu, fever, diabetes, and pathological changes of the thyroid gland. Headaches can also arise in connection with digestive disorders. Relaxing or sleeping and taking of antacids relieves stomach ache and headache.

There are several theories as to how the headache is formed. Some suggest that the irritation of pain receptors is influenced by stress, by increased muscle tension, or dilation of blood vessels. Other studies show pathological changes, particularly the serotonin balance disorder.

Important in diagnosis is the character and localization of pain, occurrence of the disease in the family, exclusion of other diseases, blood tests, electrolytes (sodium and chloride, bicarbonate, calcium, magnesium), analysis of renal function (creatinine), erythrocyte sedimentation rate, etc. Treatment depends on the type of pain. Mostly stronger analgesics or painkillers are used. Other possibilities are, for example, oxygen therapy, relaxation, vitamins, minerals, physical activity (aerobic exercise), or a change in eating habits.

CHAPTER 3

AN IN DEPTH LOOK AT MIGRAINES

Everyone who suffers a strong headache often believes that it is a migraine. However, doctors distinguish between what is a "typical" and "atypical" form of the disease. Sometimes even a lack of headache itself is an atypical migraine.

1. Pain in the face

Many patients with atypical migraine are complaining of facial pain, ranging from mild to strong and difficult conditions. The pain may be constant and the most common is located around the eyes. The face may also be sensitive to the touch, although pain can be decreased by applying pressure or massage to facial reflex points.

2. Abdominal Problems

Although headache is most commonly associated with migraine, abdominal cramps are also quite frequent. Cramps are similar to menstrual ones. Women have symptoms of nausea and vomiting.

3. Neurological effects

Atypical migraine can often take a very scary turn. In some cases, neurological effects are also observed. Extreme cases caused damages such as numbness and paralysis of the arm or even the entire body. This effect lasts for no more than a few minutes without permanent damage. Some patients also reported tingling on one side of the body, which took a short period of time (in minutes) and then the pain decreased.

4. Eye disorders

Visual disorders are quite common with atypical migraine. Patients often report an "aura", a sort of rainbow color in the visual field. There are sometimes flashes of light and flicker in peripheral vision.

Atypical migraine symptoms are decreased in a cool, dark and quiet room with medicines containing the active ingredient. Chronic migraine should be treated with drugs that function to compensate chemicals in the brain. Migraine belongs to the group of so-called functional headaches. It affects people of working age from twenty-five to fifty-five years of life. Triggering factors may be stress, physical exertion, change of weather (air pressure), lack of sleep, fatigue, hormonal and other factors as well.

Neurologists recommend to rest in a dark room, and adequate drinking of water. In the early stages only commonly available painkillers are used, but if this does not bring the desired effect, the patient should consult with a doctor. It is a diagnosis that should certainly be monitored and treated by a specialist. Most migraine sufferers have migraine without "aura", but for some patients it is an indication of attack, which is manifested by various transient neurological symptoms, mostly visual. It may be different flashes of light, scintillating images, but also sensitivity to smells and touch, numbness or speech disorder, dizziness, double vision, noise in the ears or temporary hearing disorders.

A migraine headache can sometimes be confused with a certain type of bleeding. It can be bleeding from a blood vessel, which may crack and cause headache. This is significantly unusual in headache and some people even hear the rupture in the head. Rupture may be provoked by sneeze, cough, or rebounds may also arise out of nowhere during jogging. Such headaches can be confused with migraine attack. But the patient, who knows the migraine attacks, would be able to distinguish these pains. If anyone else had such an experience, then it cannot be mistaken. In the tension-type headaches, the patient has the feeling that his head is going to be crushed. So it is not pulsing migraine pain, but pressure pain, which often tend to be associated with a feeling of nausea. They are often the result of long work by the computer, so it is important to interrupt the work, give yourself a few minutes of massage and relax nuchal muscles.

It is not a life-threatening pain, but they tend to be frequent and tend to be combined with migraine headaches. Then we can talk about mixed headaches, which are complicated and in this case should be treated as both diagnoses. They are common in sensitive people who are often overworked. It is connected with anxiety, depression, sleep disorders and tension. Quite a few women know the headaches associated with the onset of menstruation. These headaches arise due to hormonal changes. Unambiguous help is problematic. During this period, a woman should avoid food allergens. It is also important to take the medicine at the onset of the first symptoms. Cold compresses and rest in a quiet and darkened room also help. Headaches may also show during hormonal contraceptive use and there are also other side effects such as vomiting, breast tenderness, mood changes, or weight gain.

Women with migraine who use hormonal contraceptives may present with an increased risk of stroke in relation to other risk factors such as smoking. Children can also suffer migraines, but the diagnosis is problematic, since the symptoms cannot be well described by them. Medicine of an herbal origin is used for treatment.

Headaches tend to occur to children in relation to hormonal changes during puberty. In such cases, neurologists recommend to increase magnesium or give analgesics. A common reason is, for example, stress at school, without having to be a migraine. It tends to be mostly tension-type headaches due to muscle tension. Headaches may also result from food and beverages. Most common can be chocolate, cheese, nuts, onion, vinegar, dressings, soy sauce, liver, or seafood. Pain can occur even after the use of certain vitamins - A, for example, and similarly after the ingestion of vitamin B6, selenium, or iodine. It is usual also to talk about the so-called "Chinese restaurant syndrome", when the headache is induced by substance MSG (monosodium glutamate). Headaches can be caused by hunger, as well, resulting from low blood sugar and vasodilation. This kind of headache should disappear after ingestion of food containing mainly sugars and proteins.

Pain may also result from excessive alcohol consumption, which causes constriction of blood vessels, brain edema and dysregulation of water and electrolyte metabolism. If the person is a coffee drinker with regular intake of caffeine, headache may appear in case he/she missed a regular cup of coffee.

CHAPTER 4

NATURAL WAYS TO CURE A HEADACHE

Currently, we are spending huge money on drugs and we use them like candy. We know this is not exactly the best solution. There are many ways to beat the headache without pills. How to do it? Headaches are a common problem of many people. Whether it is stress, lack of sleep, or other causes, headache can truly worsen life. However, while searching for quick and easy assistance in the form of some pills, first there are a few natural ways rather than a chemical weapon cocktail of drugs.

1. Mint tea
This herb has a positive effect on the digestive system, and headaches are often associated with problems in this area. One cup of mint tea should bring relief.

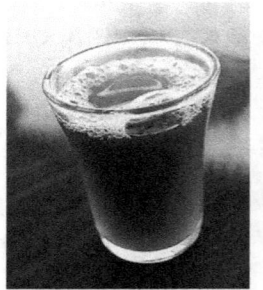

2. Peppermint oil on the forehead
Many studies have shown that peppermint essential oil helps, as well. It has healing powers and it stimulates receptors in the skin.

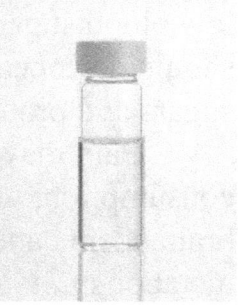

3. Coffee

Sometimes it is recommended to drink a cup of coffee when the first symptoms of headaches are starting to show. Caffeine causes the blood vessels to expand, and headaches will disappear. Called "coffee bomb" , 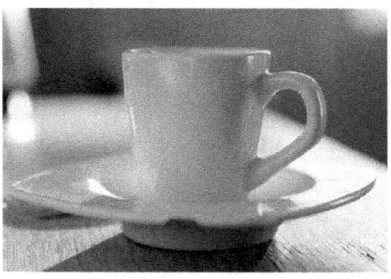 this can be effective for people who do not drink coffee regularly. Then it will help to pour a drop of lemon into coffee. Caffeine blocks the creation of a special enzyme that is responsible for causing the pain.

4. Ginger

Ginger can be great help for headaches. For stopping the pain of headaches, patient should cut up a piece of ginger root, place it in hot water and let steep for a few minutes. It is possible then to remove the ginger pieces or leave it in a cup and drink it slowly. A good tip is to add a little honey and lemon juice. Ginger has a 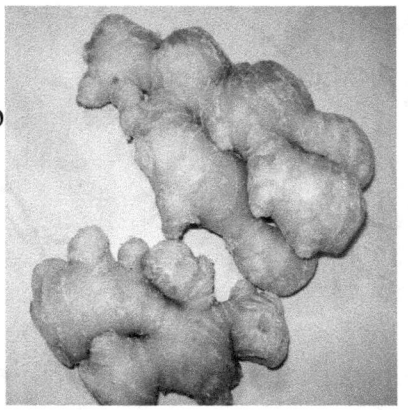 number of positive effects on our health; for example, it helps with colds.

5. Cold or warm compress

According to some experts, warm or cold compresses are no science-based "medicine" against headaches. On the other hand, the truth is that many times it really helps. Depending on the type of headache as well as the person him or herself, it may bring relief via cold compress or warm. The patient has to find a quiet place to lay, put on his/her forehead a cotton diaper soaked in cold or warm water for a moment and then relax. Closing of eyes will also help to decrease the pain.

Warm compress – 50% of people have a headache because of pulled muscles in the cervical spine. Pain reduction can be achieved by aligning the neck of the bottle with hot water. After some time, the muscle relaxes and headache passes.

Cold compress - A good assistant is also a cold compress on the eyes and forehead. This helps with headaches and fever.

6. Drink!

Often a headache is caused by insufficient intake of fluids. If the person do not keep up fluid intake, his/her body does not immediately start to demonstrate dehydration, but headaches are one of the symptoms of lack of fluids. When the person feels that headache is coming, he/she should quickly take a drink of clean water or fruit or vegetable juice. Sometimes it helps, sometimes it cannot be saved by only a glass of water. But give it a try.

7. Pencil in the teeth

A slightly strange old wives' tale is to insert a pencil into the mouth, between upper and lower teeth. Simply take one pencil, put it between teeth and hold (it should not be chewed or somehow strongly clenched). This method looks strange, but it is often very effective.

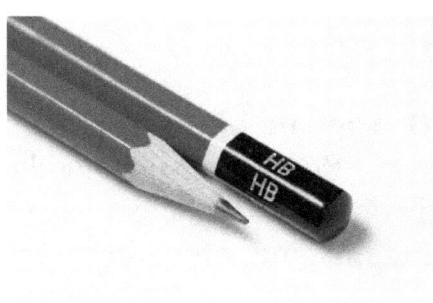

Photo by Dmgerman

8. The miracle named oak bark

Its main active ingredient is salicin, of which a synthetic form appears in aspirin. When it is placed in hot water and strained, it is possible to drink it as a tea.

9. Release at work

Photo By Jun'ichiro Seyama

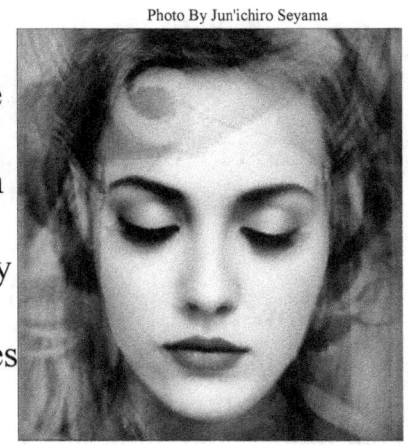

Long hours in front of the screen of the computer can also be a cause of headaches. Improper seating and poor head carriage can cause a more long-lasting headache. At work, it is good to try to take a break. Exercise with the head and do not forget that the eyes also need to rest.

10. Massage of temples

Thumbs can be put on temples and massage has to be provided very softly in circular movements. Yoga also helps.

11. Cinema in the head

Sometimes it is good just to lie on your back, close your eyes, and imagine something pleasant.

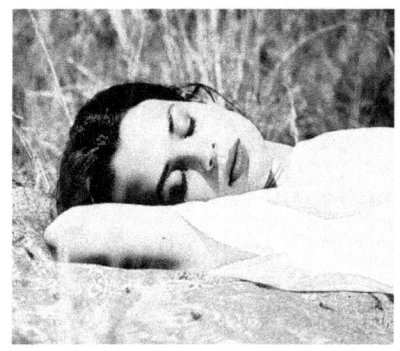

Photo By Kris Krog

12. Butterbur medical

This herb is priceless. Tea can be cooked from fresh and dried forms.

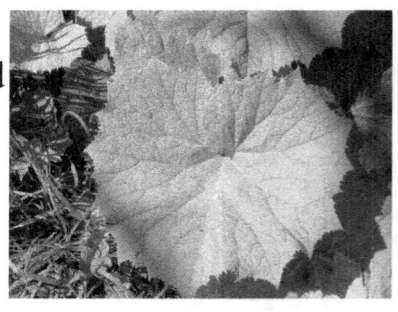

If none of the above tips help, there is a time for a pill. Unfortunately, even this is not a guaranteed method and it always takes a while for the effects of any medication to kick in.

13. Know the Cause!

It is necessary to know why the you have a headache. The cause may be the already mentioned primary or secondary headache (stress, premenstrual period or lack of sleep, etc).
If symptoms persist, see a doctor.

CHAPTER 5

HOW TO AVOID HEADACHES

According to a recent Belgian study, a daily given dosage of 400 mg of riboflavin reduced the frequency (but not the severity and duration) of chronic migraine attacks by about one third. The study reported that riboflavin may be useful for patients suffering from an average of four migraine attacks per month. Certain foods and beverages, particularly those containing compounds known as amines, can be considered the most infamous cause of migraine. If someone has a migraine, he/she should try to avoid mature cheese, onions, pickled vegetables, nuts, smoked meat, red wine, beer, sour cream, fresh sourdough bread, citrus fruits, tomatoes, eggs and caffeinated beverages. These are often the cause of the seizures.

Traditionally, chocolate can cause migraine, but according to new studies, this is not completely true. The inclusion of fish, rich in omega-3 fatty acids, may help to prevent migraines. Omega-3 fatty acids alter the chemical substances contained in the blood and reduce the risk of vascular spasm associated with migraine.

What are other possible causes of headaches? Sudden change of weather - many people are not able to sufficiently adapt to the changing weather conditions. The body may respond with changes in blood pressure, dizziness, circulatory disorders and sleep disorders, and also headaches.

Very tired eyes – the head may hurt even more if the person reads in low light, or when he/she stares long hours at a television or computer screen.

Psychological stress - if the patient is under long-term stress and has anxiety or is in a depressed mood, headaches often result. The pain is described as dull pressure in the temples or the whole head.

Illness from colds and flu - pain in the face, especially the forehead, is often an indication of inflammation of the side and frontal sinuses.

What is interesting is that the treating of headache by aspirin or other analgesics may counteract the natural ability of the body to relieve pain.

CONCLUSION

Headaches and migraine is not just a problem of hypochondriacs and hysterical women. This is a real disease, which is also described in the International Classification of Diseases. Headache as a symptom of the disease may be accompanied by simple diseases, but on the other hand, it may also be a life-threatening condition. No headache should be underestimated. Pain warns that something with the body is not alright. Acute pain is usually a signal for indicating imbalance of the workings of the body. So it is a sign of disease.

Perception and pain management are concerned with sensory nerve fibers and their endings. The brain itself does not have these fibers, and therefore the brain is not able to experience pain. Headaches as known by most people have their origins outside the cranial cavity. Skin, muscles, ligaments, surface of bones, mucous membranes, eyes and teeth are richly interwoven with sensitive nerve fibers and these can be a source of pain. Primary headaches that occur with diabetes, obesity, high blood pressure, heart attacks, or strokes are sometimes called "civilization diseases".

93 percent of men and 99 percent of women suffer from diverse types of headaches and migraines. Signs of migraine can occur at any age. Seizures usually begin in childhood or adolescence. More often it affects boys, but the ratio moves "in favor" of girls at puberty. If the person suffers the headache repeatedly, a doctor should be consulted. Probably he will say that everything is fine, but if not, he will send the patient for further examination.

Other Books By Dr Brad Turner

Aromatherapy The Beginner's Guide:

Frankincense. Peppermint. Eucalyptus. Lemongrass. Lavender. Who knew that these are five of the must have essential oils? Dr. Brad Turner does—and we are blessed that he's chosen to share his knowledge and expertise in his latest book, ESSENTIAL OILS. So much has been written about using oils: as cures for everything from toothaches to acne; aromatherapy and even taken internally for whatever reason is popular that day.. To our own peril, we've discovered much of this information is false. Dr. Turner gains our trust immediately with his treatise: never ingest these essential oils. And that's the beginning of an author/reader relationship that will stand the test of time…and information, because Dr. Turner tells the truth. And that's the way we like it!

Lose Belly Fat Without Exercise

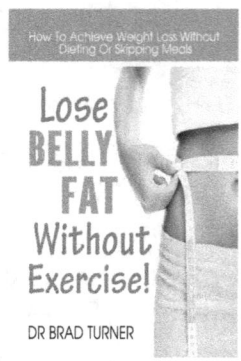

Dr Brad Turner's Lose Belly Fat Without Exercise is an easy to follow guide which gives you the important information you need to give you a jump start to a vibrant, radiant and sexy new you!
If you are tired of counting calories, fat grams and points and or have lost your motivation with crash course Exercise programs and are tired of diets that just do not work, then this book is for you.